Environment of Care Sample Report to Leadership

By Steven A. MacArthur

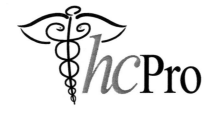

Steven A. MacArthur, Contributing Author
Cara Connors, Senior Managing Editor
Lauren Rubenzahl, Proofreader
Jackie Diehl Singer, Graphic Artist
Paul Singer, Layout Artist
Jean St. Pierre, Creative Director
Shane Katz, Cover Designer
Bob Croce, Group Publisher
Suzanne Perney, Publisher

Advice given is general. Readers should consult professional counsel for specific legal, ethical, or clinical questions.

Arrangements can be made for quantity discounts. For more information, contact:

HCPro, Inc.
P.O. Box 1168
Marblehead, MA 01945
Telephone: 800/650-6787 or 781/639-1872
Fax: 781/639-2982
E-mail: *customerservice@hcpro.com*

Visit HCPro at its World Wide Web sites:
www.hcpro.com, www.hcmarketplace.com, www.accreditinfo.com

CONTENTS

About the Contributing Author

Steven A. MacArthur

Steven A. MacArthur is a safety consultant in the accreditation and regulatory compliance division of The Greeley Company, a division of HCPro, Inc., in Marblehead, MA. He conducts on-site safety assessments and educational programs as well as regulatory survey preparation for safety leaders. He develops comprehensive programs related to the environment of care (EC) and various other consulting/professional services, including interim staffing.

He consults and lectures on the Joint Commission on Accreditation of Healthcare Organizations' (JCAHO) EC standards and on guidelines and regulations from the Occupational Safety and Health Administration (OSHA), the Environmental Protection Agency, the Department of Environmental Protection, and the Department of Public Health. He works with hospitals, physician practices, ambulatory care, long-term care, home care, and behavioral-health facilities in preparing for and responding to JCAHO accreditation and OSHA compliance surveys.

He authored the book *Preparing for Mass Casualty Incidents: Hospital Readiness for Biological, Chemical, and Radiological Disasters* and serves as both the contributing editor of the newsletter *Briefings on Hospital Safety* and an editorial advisor to the newsletter *Healthcare Security and Emergency Management.*

He has worked in the fields of healthcare environmental services and safety for 25 years.

PRODUCE AN ANNUAL **EC** REPORT THAT'S CURRENT, CONCISE, AND MEANINGFUL

Meet both leadership's and Joint Commission expectations

As a hospital safety professional, you find yourself with an ever-increasing workload. Churning out a concise, readable, and comprehensive environment of care (EC) annual report to hospital leaders each year is part of that responsibility.

The Joint Commission on Accreditation of Healthcare Organizations (JCAHO) views this report as one of the cornerstones of your EC program. As part of the new survey process, surveyors will conduct the EC section of the survey based on what they learn from reviewing your annual EC program evaluation, your EC/safety committee minutes, and your *Statement of Conditions*. As no other documents are in the official "review" list for survey, the focus on, and the importance of your annual evaluations has never been greater.

In a survey of healthcare safety professionals conducted in early 2004, about 70% of survey respondents said JCAHO surveyors discussed standards EC.9.10, which calls for monitoring of the EC, and EC.9.20, which calls for identifying EC issues. HCPro, Inc., the publisher of this workbook, conducted the survey.

"The focus of the EC portion [of the survey] was how risks in the EC are managed, how opportunities are identified, and how improvements are made, especially as a function over time," answered one respondent to a question about survey hotspots.

Another respondent said JCAHO surveyors were "very interested" in the hospital's monitoring of EC indicators for the seven performance areas.

Here's help

We've created this workbook to help EC and safety leaders produce their annual EC reports to meet both leaders' and JCAHO expectations. In this section, we'll discuss the elements that go into producing those reports.

If you belong to a healthcare system, member facilities can tailor the charts we've provided to their own safety programs. We've also provided you with tips to help you present your report to hospital leadership.

Although some goals may be obvious—such as items requested by administration or regulatory requirements—others may not be immediately apparent. By following the template in this workbook when planning for the year, safety committees will focus on areas that they might otherwise forget.

Refocus your plans to satisfy the JCAHO

When planning and completing the report, remember that the *JCAHO's Shared Visions—New Pathways®* process has changed how surveyors will review your EC program.

Surveyors will expect you to identify improvements based on committee activities and flesh them out into program goals through annual evaluations. The days of using the annual evaluations to report on process activity are disappearing. Now the focus is squarely on management of risk and identifying measurable opportunities for improvement.

Surveyors will track goals, activities, indicators, etc., back to EC-committee meeting minutes, so the minutes have to be in good shape before you can reasonably expect to evaluate your program.

Make sure minutes are complete in that they both bring up and resolve issues. If, for example, the minutes note an upswing in thefts over the holidays, they should also document what action you've taken to address this issue.

How to use the forms

After you've reviewed the year as captured in the committee minutes, it's time to create a report for your governing board or leaders. Use the templates in this workbook to cover each of the seven JCAHO-required management plans—safety, life safety, security, utilities, medical equipment, hazardous materials, and emergency management.

Each form describes the scope of the program and includes a grid you can use to list your annual objectives, associated performance indicators, the effectiveness of the program, and future recommendations. In the workbook, we've filled out the forms using a sample case study to show you how to use them. They appear blank on the CD-ROM so you can enter your own information.

Identify and document priorities at the beginning of the year. If the priorities change during the year (and that's a very good possibility, unless your crystal ball is working exceptionally well), you'll have a record of what you'd set out to accomplish—a record you can use as both a means of evaluation of the current year and a planning tool for future cycles.

For example, if the problem of stolen or lost materials creates a major expense, it may become the basis for a performance-improvement project or a change in policy. As the year wears on, that problem may fall by the wayside as the hospital devotes resources to issues that more immediately affect patient or employee safety. But the data will exist to remind the safety committee that the problem of stolen and lost materials needs attention when time permits.

Six tips for a smooth and efficient leadership report

Deliver your environment of care annual report to leaders in a quick but comprehensive presentation with these tips:

1. **Make it clean.** Make your report easy to understand with easy-to-follow sections and quick reference points so leaders can quickly see whether the facility achieved its goals.
2. **Get to the point.** You will have a limited amount of leadership's time. If serious problems exist that you want to call to its attention, put these problems at the front of the report so they don't get lost in the discussion of lesser goals or problems.
3. **Make it simple.** Don't make your report so brief that it doesn't say anything but keep it as simple as possible.
4. **Include accomplishments and carryovers.** Discuss which goals you achieved and which items you want to carry over to next year. Leaders will appreciate knowing there is an ongoing process that doesn't begin and end with the start of each new year.
5. **Sing your own praises.** Don't be afraid to highlight projects you did well. If you don't do it in the annual evaluation to leaders, when will you do it? Leaders need to know about your accomplishments and the value of the hard work performed by the safety committee.
6. **Seek feedback.** The Joint Commission on Accreditation of Healthcare Organizations wants to see that leaders received reports from the safety committee, but also that they responded in a way that makes them understand their role in the safety program.

Also be sure to consider the always-fluid federal, state, and local regulatory scene when choosing objectives. For example, if an objective is to improve handwashing technique, set up a program to achieve hand-hygiene compliance.

When your hospital accomplishes a goal in one area—for example, creating an improved policy—it might trigger a goal for another area, such as employee knowledge. The teams that regularly review each area of the hospital may then focus on the new policy when questioning staff.

A deficiency in awareness of or adherence to new policies could prompt greater educational efforts and changes in staffing so the policy can be carried out more effectively.

In addition to the seven EC-management plans, this workbook contains a template for subjects that aren't strictly JCAHO issues.

For example, you could highlight workers' compensation in the safety section. You could cover other employee-health issues, such as exposure-control plans, by creating similar plans for them. Don't forget clinics and offices not located at the hospital—they may have their own issues for which you want to develop plans.

A note about indicators

Surveyors don't want to see your organization batting 1,000 with each indicator, but rather want to find you reviewing your activities at the committee level to identify issues to monitor and improve. Need help choosing indicators? See p. 11 for a list of dos and don'ts. Also, we've included sample indicators for each of the seven areas on p. 7.

Tip: Choose indicators that can show improvement over time and show surveyors graphs depicting your performance over time, because as one survey respondent said, JCAHO surveyors "looked for historical performance to be included in annual program evaluations."

SAMPLE EC PERFORMANCE INDICATORS

Not sure which indicators to use in seeking areas to improve within the environment of care (EC)? We've compiled a list of examples for your consideration. When reviewing them, select those that are appropriate to your organization.

Safety management	Equipment management
Percentage of successful follow-up actions taken in response to hazard-surveillance deficiencies (>95%)	Percentage of compliance with preventive maintenance (PM) efforts
Number of employee needlesticks	Number of pieces of unfound/could-not-locate equipment
Number of patient elopements	Number of hazard recalls/alerts completed
Number of patient falls	Number of incident reports, user errors
Number of back injuries	Number of incident reports, damaged equipment
	Percentage of user-training attendance
Security management	**Utilities management**
Percentage of annual EC training attendance (>95%)	Percentage of compliance PMs
Number of working panic devices (100%)	Percentage of annual EC-training attendance (>95%)
Number of door-alarm batteries that are inoperable (0)	Number of elevator failures
Number of maternity false alarms	Number of elevator entrapments
Percentage of security staff training attendance	Electricity costs (reduce by 4%)
	Costs for fuel oil (reduce by 2%)
	Number of utility failures resulting in adverse patient outcomes

Hazardous material and waste management	Fire-prevention/life-safety management
Number of needlesticks as a result of inappropriate disposal	Percentage of completed life-safety code PMs
Number of spills cleaned in accordance with hospital procedure	Percentage of annual EC-training attendance
Reduction of volume of regulated waste (<12,000 lbs.)	Percentage of actual fire emergencies
Number of radiation exposures	Number of false alarms in construction areas
Number of mercury devices removed from the facility	Number of first responders attending drills
Number of mercury devices remaining in the facility	
Emergency management	
Number of timely callbacks to emergency pages (7 minutes response time)	
Number of fully stocked disaster carts (100%)	
Percentage of annual EC-training attendance (>95%)	
Percentage of leadership trained on incident-command system	

TRACK YOUR EC PROGRESS WITH THESE SAMPLE PERFORMANCE INDICATORS

Listed below are examples of performance indicators you can use to monitor and measure your environment of care (EC) program efforts.

Remember to include the following in your performance indicator sets:
- The indicator or measure used.
- The data, the source of the data, and the overall population of items, people, or activities being sampled or measured.
- The data-collection interval. This interval includes the frequency with which you collect the data, such as quarterly, and how often you analyze it.
- Sample sizes. The sample should contain at least 10% of the population (5% for groups or populations over 500), or a minimum of 30 staff observed. Some samples will cover 100% of the population. Others will include random samples (for large groups of data).
- Reporting format. This refers to the format in which you will present the information, generally through graphs. Examples include control or run charts, bar charts, and scatter diagrams.

Please remember that the following indicators do not necessarily reflect a specific JCAHO standard; they merely represent the types of things you can look at in your program. Identify goals that are achievable but challenging. Look carefully at those compliance percentages. Don't set the bar too low or too high. Don't be afraid to reflect your organization's experience—it is an important consideration when adopting your performance indicators.

Here are sample performance indicators for you to think about:

1. Safety
- **People**
  - Staff knowledge: Percentage of staff's correct answers to defined questions
- **Equipment**
  - Readiness: Availability of personal protective equipment (PPE) for staff who require it as observed during inspections and other rounds (perform 30 observations, or observe 10% of your organization's staff)

- **Administration**
  - Percentage of areas scheduled for inspection that were inspected on time
  - Percentage of staff who use PPE when applicable (10% of population, or a minimum of 30 staff observed)

2. Security
- **People**
  - Staff knowledge: Percentage of correct answers to defined questions
- **Equipment**
  - Percentage of alarms and access-control equipment in sensitive areas that function as designed during testing and drills
- **Administration**
  - Percentage of staff wearing badges where indicated

3. Hazardous materials and wastes
- **People**
  - Staff knowledge: Percentage of correct answers to defined questions
- **Equipment**
  - Percentage of containers with appropriate labels
  - Percentage of carts used to transport hazardous wastes with proper covers
- **Administration**
  - Waste reduction: Weight of infectious waste shipped (use manifest weight), showing decrease in amount over time

4. Emergency management
- **People**
  - Staff knowledge: Percentage of correct answers to defined questions
- **Equipment**
  - Emergency-equipment readiness: Percentage of equipment ready, percentage of medication and supplies found to be up-to-date during regular inspections
- **Administration**
  - Percentage of problems identified during drills or activations that are

monitored and determined to be corrected

5. Life-safety management

- **People**
    - Staff knowledge: Percentage of correct answers to defined questions
- **Equipment**
    - A sample of fire extinguishers that have undergone inspection, are in appropriate condition, and appropriate location
- **Administration**
    - Fire drills are observed in a certain percentage of occupied areas in addition to a location adjacent to (above, below, diagonal) the primary location of the drill

6. Medical equipment

- **People**
    - Staff knowledge: Percentage of correct answers to defined questions
    - Staff who use life-critical equipment are able to describe emergency procedures
- **Equipment**
    - Percentage of preventive maintenance activities and inspections completed in a timely manner
- **Administration**
    - Percentage of employees who use medical equipment who are clinically evaluated for competence

7. Utility management

- **People**
    - Staff knowledge: Percentage of correct answers to defined questions
- **Equipment**
    - Percentage of preventive maintenance activities and inspections completed in a timely manner
- **Administration**
    - Percentage of employees who service utility-systems equipment deemed competent during their evaluations

Do these EC sample goals apply to your hospital?
Consider using them in your EC program

If you're stumped on selecting goals for your environment of care (EC) program, look over the sample goals below. Choose any that apply to your organization and would help resolve existing problems or improve systems, practices, or processes:

- **Safety management**
  - Track appropriate follow-up actions to hazard-surveillance deficiencies (=/>98% completion rate)
  - Reduce workers' compensation expenses through workers' compensation team (negative trend)
  - Reduce needlesticks through blood and body-fluid performance-improvement team (negative trend)
  - Review and revise ergonomics program

- **Security management**
  - Conduct a minimum of two infant-abduction drills
  - Reduce maternity security system faults—e.g., false alarms, etc. (negative trend)
  - Conduct a minimum of two facility-lockdown drills
  - Test security alarm-system components quarterly (=/>95% operation)

- **Hazardous materials and waste management**
  - Implement material safety data sheet (MSDS) on-demand system
  - Initiate quarterly testing of MSDS availability (100% availability)
  - Continue focus on reducing mercury and other hazardous materials
  - Track the number of hazardous-materials spills cleaned in accordance with protocol (100% compliance)
  - Track the number of radiation exposures (0 incidents)

- **Emergency management**
  - Conduct a minimum of two emergency drill activations (one that involves communitywide participation)
  - Revise hazard-vulnerability analysis to reflect current conditions
  - Track the percentage of annual EC-training attendance (=/>97% compliance)

- **Life-safety management**
  - Conduct an interim life safety measures (ILSM) assessment for each component of construction project (100% compliance)
  - Track the completion percentage of weekly ILSM inspection activities (100% compliance)
  - Track the percentage of life safety system preventive-maintenance (PM) activities (=/>95% completion rate)
  - Track the completion of percentage of follow-up on emergency-drill deficiencies (100% completion rate)

- **Medical equipment management**
  - Track the completion percentage of PM activities (=/>95% completion rate)
  - Track the completion of percentage of corrective-maintenance activities (=/>95% completion rate)
  - Comply with National Patient Safety Goal #5 regarding free-flow pumps
  - Comply with National Patient Safety Goal #6 regarding clinical alarms

- **Utilities management**
  - Track the completion of percentage of preventive-maintenance activities (=/>95% completion rate)
  - Review all utilities disruptions by tracking the percentage associated with PM activity deficiencies (whether disruption was preventable: <1% incident rate)
  - Track the number of utilities disruptions resulting in adverse patient outcomes (0 incidents)

CONSIDER THESE TIPS ABOUT CHOOSING INDICATORS

Here's a quick rundown of the dos and don'ts of choosing indicators.

Do
- choose indicators that show improvements over time
- select indicators based on repeatable activity, such as observations
- choose issues central to the function of the program
- select issues of interest to two management levels above you

Know these three EC survey hot spots and how to avoid them

Show Joint Commission on Accreditation of Healthcare Organizations' (JCAHO) surveyors evidence of your environment of care (EC) compliance efforts by avoiding these survey pitfalls:

- **Failure to complete the annual evaluation for each of the seven EC sections.** Make sure the individual(s) responsible for each of the seven sections of the EC complete the annual evaluation. Although it's easy to overlook this requirement, it's the basis for your performance-improvement program, and surveyors will check to make sure you've completed it.

- **Failure to identify one performance-improvement activity in the EC and to make the recommendation to organization leadership.** The JCAHO expects you to identify at least one performance-improvement initiative in the EC program every year and make a recommendation to the organization's leaders. The improvement project can pertain to any one of the seven EC functions and can even take place as a part of your normal work responsibilities. This does not mean, however, that the organization's leaders have to adopt the recommendation, particularly if it involves a costly allocation of resources (remember that they write the checks, so it is absolutely within their purview to table a recommendation that doesn't fit into their strategic initiatives). However, if it is something you can accomplish as a function of the program, make sure that you both take credit for your work and document the process and results.

- **Failure to meet on an appropriately regular basis.** Meetings form the foundation of your annual report to leaders by being the source of performance-improvement projects and a forum for reviewing outcomes. Although the JCAHO doesn't require a separate safety or EC committee, it's easy to forget the requirement that says to have a multidisciplinary group meet regularly to discuss EC-related issues—in many instances, committee members are involved in other activities and just don't have a chance to meet. Keep copies of each meeting's agenda, minutes, and any information distributed (e.g., reports, etc.) to provide validation to JCAHO surveyors that the multidisciplinary team has met and discussed outcomes at appropriate intervals. Remember that although the standards do allow meetings to be held more or less frequently than bimonthly, as long as the frequency is supported by current hospital experience and safety-committee approval, ongoing justification of meeting frequency is dependent on a satisfactory annual evaluation of performance. If you're not meeting at least bimonthly, be prepared to defend your decision during survey.

SAMPLE CASE STUDY: HOW TO USE THE ENCLOSED FORMS IN YOUR FACILITY

To show you how to use the forms in this workbook, we've created a case study based on different facilities' environment of care (EC) management plans.

The intent of this case study is to provide a glimpse into the penultimate product of the EC-management process: the annual evaluation of the program. From this product springs improvement opportunities. The evaluation begins on day one of your annual cycle and continues through day 365. It reflects a comprehensive summary of the processes and activities that constitute a successful—or unsuccessful—EC program.

If you've evaluated your program and not found anything to improve, you're either looking at the wrong items or you're not examining your program with a critical eye. There's always room for improvement.

The management form is the basis for your communication with both your organization's leaders and the overall organization. For those of you in more complex organizations, remember to include in your form satellite facilities that operate under your umbrella. Surveyors have become more attentive to integrating risk management in all environments. And after all, that's what you're evaluating: the management of your organization's environmental risks.

Pick pertinent performance indicators

For the purposes of this example, we've chosen performance indicators that are more generic than those you'd probably pick for your organization. However, these indicators are appropriate to the intent of this process as well as to the applicable standards, so you may want to use them if you need help getting your process started. Each of these indicators has been presented during surveys in the last 12 months.

Identifying performance indicators in any organization is by no means a cookie-cutter endeavor. The key indicators used to evaluate performance in your EC-management program should be a useful mix of process-oriented indicators and outcome-oriented measures.

Choose indicators that are meaningful and offer ways to measure success or lack thereof. Where possible, show trends and analyses of issues identified during the course of your evaluation. Successful performance is good, but more valuable is understanding why your performance was successful. With this knowledge, you can ensure the integrity and ongoing performance of your program.

Last words

As a final reminder, Joint Commission on Accreditation of Healthcare Organizations' standards require you to use only one performance indicator for each of the seven EC functions and communicate only one performance-improvement recommendation to leaders. (Note that our case study reflects a more far-reaching program evaluation.)

"Useful" and "meaningful" are the watchwords for what you choose to evaluate. Don't monitor the basic items you're supposed to be doing, unless you have a significant issue. For example, surveyors expect you to conduct the appropriate number of drills and surveillance rounds, so don't monitor the drills and rounds. Instead, evaluate the items you look at during those activities to identify improvement opportunities or to validate that your systems are intact and function appropriately.

The annual evaluation is not a means to an end; it's both the means and the end.

If you have difficulty justifying what you're monitoring, reexamine your choices. Are they useful and meaningful? If they pass those criteria, you can successfully navigate any survey process.

Leadership response to the annual evaluation of the EC program

The annual evaluation of the environment of care (EC) program is prepared for hospital leaders in compliance with Joint Commission on Accreditation of Healthcare Organizations (JCAHO) standard EC __. The format includes narrative summaries, financial data, and performance indicators to provide a comprehensive and concise report that facilitates informed decision-making.

In compliance with the intent of standard EC __, a documented response to the _____ committee, which oversees the environment of care, is appreciated. Thank you.

Leadership response (select one):

_____ Hospital leaders have received this report from the _____ committee and concur with the recommendations of that committee.

_____ Hospital leaders have received the report from the _____ committee and would like additional information on the following items: _____
_____
_____

_____ Hospital leaders have received the report from the _____ committee and recommend the following: _____
_____
_____

Signatures:

_____
Safety officer

_____
Committee chair

_____
Administrative representative

cc: ___ Medical-policy committee
    ___ Quality-assurance committee
    ___ Risk-management committee
    ___ Infection-control committee

[Your facility's name]
Environment of care management program
Annual evaluation of program

January 1, 2003–December 31, 2003

SAFETY MANAGEMENT

Scope of program

[Your facility's name] safety program provides patients, staff, and visitors with an environment free from recognized safety and health hazards both by promoting staff activities that reduce the risk of injuries and illnesses and by fostering an accident- and injury-preventive culture. The safety-management program and management plan have been reviewed for content and scope. The safety-management plan was revised to reflect current (2004) standards and expectations.

Performance of program

The following chart shows the program objectives, the indicator(s) measured to achieve the stated objective(s), the effectiveness of the program, and future recommendations.

Indicators	Objectives	Performance (2001–2003)
Staff knowledge of unsafe/hazard-condition reporting (response to query during rounds, emergency drills)	>/= 95% staff can articulate means of reporting unsafe/ hazardous conditions	2001—New indicator for 2002 2002—91.7% staff responded appropriately 2003—94% staff responded appropriately **Process stable with improvement; objective not met—continue to monitor**
Safe lifting technique (staff can articulate/ demonstrate during rounds)	>/= 95% staff articulated/ demonstrated appropriate knowledge 2002—New indicator for 2003	2003—92.3% staff responded appropriately **Process stable w/improvement; objective not met—continue to monitor**

Effectiveness of program/recommendations for improvement

The scope and performance of [your facility's name] safety program is determined to have been effective to the extent called for in the 2003 management plan. This determination is based on a comprehensive evaluation of the safety management program and its objectives and the monitoring of applicable performance indicators and performance relative to objective goals, with improvement areas identified for ongoing monitoring. Additionally, no critical failure modes were identified as a function of [your facility's name] incident-reporting system. The following improvement opportunities have been identified for 2004:

Improvement opportunity/objective	Indicator/measure
Staff knowledge of hazard reporting (continue monitoring)	>/= 95% staff queried can articulate/ demonstrate knowledge
Staff knowledge of safe lifting techniques (continue monitoring)	>/= 95% staff queried can articulate/ demonstrate knowledge
Maintain safety of environment for staff	Reduction of workers' compensation expenses

[Your facility's name]
Environment of care management program
Annual evaluation of program

January 1, 2003–December 31, 2003

LIFE-SAFETY MANAGEMENT

Scope of program

[Your facility's name] life-safety management program ensures a functionally safe environment in and around the hospital and protects patients, staff, and visitors from fire and the products of combustion. [Your facility's name] life-safety management program and management plan have been reviewed for content and scope. [Your facility's name] life-safety management plan was revised to reflect current (2004) standards and expectations.

Performance of program

The following chart shows the program objectives, the indicator(s) measured to achieve the stated objective(s), the effectiveness of the program, and future recommendations.

Indicators	Objectives	Performance (2001–2003)
Compliance rate of preventive-maintenance (PM) activities for all life-safety systems inventory	>/= 98% compliance rate for PM of inventory components	2001—97% compliance 2002—98.5 % compliance 2003—100% compliance **Process stable; objective met**
Staff knowledge of facility's fire plan in response to queries during rounds and drills	>/= 98% of staff queried can articulate/demonstrate knowledge of fire plan	2001—95% compliance 2002—99% compliance 2003—97% compliance **Process not stable; objective not met**

Effectiveness of program/recommendations for improvement

The scope and performance of [your facility's name] life- and fire-safety program is determined to have been effective based on the 2003 management plan. This determination is based on a comprehensive evaluation of the life- and fire-safety management program and its objectives and monitoring of applicable performance indicators and performance relative to objective goals, with improvement areas identified for ongoing monitoring. The deficit in staff knowledge of the fire plan was potentially the result of increased use of per diem staff. We will review the orientation process of per diem staff to ensure appropriate content as well as timeliness of education. Additionally, no critical failure modes were identified as a function of [your facility's name] incident-reporting system. The following improvement opportunities have been identified for 2004:

Improvement opportunity/objective	Indicator/measure
Correct all deficiencies identified during emergency drills	100% completion rate for correcting deficiencies
Conduct interim life safety measures (ILSM) assessment for all construction/renovation projects	100% compliance rate for ILSM assessment and implementation
Per diem staff knowledge of fire plan	100% of per diem staff to receive fire-safety training within two weeks of hire

[Your facility's name]
Environment of care management program
Annual evaluation of program

January 1, 2003–December 31, 2003

EMERGENCY MANAGEMENT

Scope of program

[Your facility's name] emergency-management program ensures a safe and expedient response to any natural or manmade event that could significantly affect the need for the hospital's services or its ability to provide those services. [Your facility's name] emergency-management program and management plan have been reviewed for content and scope. The emergency-management plan was revised to reflect current (2004) standards and expectations.

Performance of program

The following chart shows the program objectives, the indicator(s) measured to achieve the stated objective(s), the effectiveness of the program, and future recommendations.

Indicators	Objectives	Performance (2001–2003)
Hazard-vulnerability analysis (HVA) conducted, drill scenarios developed based on results	At least one exercise should reflect consideration of events identified as priorities through the HVA	2001—New indicator for 2002 2002—Yes—smallpox event 2003—Yes—mass-decontamination event **Process stable; objective met**
Continued implementation of incident command system (ICS)	Each drill critiques implementation of ICS as component of drill (100% compliance/minimum of two drills per year)	2002—New indicator for 2003 2003—100% drills—ICS implementation **Process stable; objective met—will continue to monitor**

Effectiveness of program/recommendations for improvement

The scope and performance of [your facility's name] emergency program is determined to have been effective as outlined in the 2003 management plan. This determination is based on a comprehensive evaluation of the emergency-management program and its objectives and monitoring of applicable performance indicators and the appropriate performance relative to objective goals, with improvement areas identified for ongoing monitoring. Additionally, no critical failure modes were identified as a function of the [your facility's name] incident-reporting system. The following improvement opportunities have been identified for 2004:

Improvement opportunity/objective	Indicator/measure
Implementation of ICS	100% exercises critiqued regarding ICS implementation
Staff participation in emergency-management education	>/= 97% staff attend and successfully complete emergency management education

[Your facility's name]
Environment of care management program
Annual evaluation of program

January 1, 2003–December 31, 2003

SECURITY MANAGEMENT

Scope of program

[Your facility's name] security-management program maintains a system of safeguards both to provide patients, staff, and visitors with a secure environment and to protect the physical property of the facility. [Your facility's name] security-management program and management plan have been reviewed for content and scope. The security-management plan was revised to reflect current (2004) standards and expectations.

Performance of program

The following chart shows the program objectives, the indicator(s) measured to achieve the stated objective(s), the effectiveness of the program, and future recommendations.

Indicators	Objectives	Performance (2001–2003)
Staff role in infant-abduction response (staff queried during rounds, drills)	>/= 95% of staff queried can articulate/demonstrate knowledge	2001—93% staff responded appropriately 2002—95% staff responded appropriately 2003—100% staff responded appropriately **Process stable; objective met**
Staff knowledge of emergency phone number (staff queried during rounds, drills)	>/=98% of staff queried can articulate knowledge	2001—95% staff responded appropriately 2002—97% staff responded appropriately 2003—100% staff responded appropriately **Process stable; objective met**
Property incidents (stolen/missing/vandalism)	Decrease in incident occurrence rate	2001—23 incidents 2002—37 incidents 2003—28 incidents **Process not stable; will continue to monitor as well as update facilitywide risk assessment**

Effectiveness of program/recommendations for improvement

The scope and performance of [your facility's name] security program is determined to have been effective as called for in the 2003 management plan. This determination is based on a comprehensive evaluation of the security-management program and its objectives and monitoring of applicable performance indicators and performance relative to objective goals, with improvement areas identified for ongoing monitoring. Additionally, no critical failure modes were identified as a function of [your facility's name] incident-reporting system. The following improvement opportunities have been identified for 2004:

Improvement opportunity/objective	Indicator/measure
Continue monitoring of property incidents as a function of risk assessment	Continued decrease in incidents
Conduct lockdown drill of facility on all shifts	Lockdown complete <20 minutes from initiation
Monitor restraint incidents in emergency department	Decrease in episode occurrence (2001–2003); historical performance shows 25% increase

[Your facility's name]
Environment of care management program
Annual evaluation of program

January 1, 2003–December 31, 2003

HAZARDOUS MATERIALS AND WASTE MANAGEMENT

Scope of program

[Your facility's name] hazardous-materials and waste-management program ensures that hazardous materials and any conditions arising from their use are handled appropriately. The program also tries to minimize risks to patients, staff, visitors, and the environment, both within and beyond the confines of the hospital, and ensure safety from the time of a material's receipt to the time of its disposal. [Your facility's name] hazardous-materials and waste-management program and management plan has been reviewed for content and scope. The hazardous-materials and waste-management plan was revised to reflect current (2004) standards and expectations.

Performance of program

The following chart shows the program objectives, the indicator(s) measured to achieve the stated objective(s), the effectiveness of the program, and future recommendations.

Indicators	Objectives	Performance (2001–2003)
Hazardous material spill/leak with staff exposure	No incidents	2001—0 incidents 2002—0 incidents 2003—0 incidents **Process stable; objective met**
Hazardous waste collection appropriately manifested and final disposition verified	100% of collection activities manifested and verified	2001—New indicator 2002—100% (review of events—100%) 2003—100% (review of events—100%) **Process stable; objective met**

Effectiveness of program/recommendations for improvement

The scope and performance of [your facility's name] hazardous-materials and wastes program is determined to have been effective as called for in the 2003 management plan. This determination is based on a comprehensive evaluation of the hazardous materials and waste-management program and its objectives; monitoring of applicable performance indicators and the appropriate performance relative to objective goals, with improvement areas identified for ongoing monitoring. Additionally, no critical failure modes were identified as a function of the [your facility's name] incident-reporting system. The following improvement opportunities identified for 2004:

Improvement opportunity/objective	Indicator/measure
Continue monitoring spill/leak incidents for exposure risks	No incidents with exposures (to staff or others)
Continue monitoring hazardous-material waste streams for regulatory compliance	100% compliance manifesting/disposition of hazardous material waste streams
Test staff knowledge of Web-based material safety data sheet (MSDS) retrieval program	>/= 95% staff can articulate/demonstrate knowledge of Web-based MSDS retrieval program (surveillance rounds)

[Your facility's name]
Environment of care management program
Annual evaluation of program

January 1, 2003–December 31, 2003

MEDICAL-EQUIPMENT MANAGEMENT

Scope of program

[Your facility's name] medical-equipment management program provides a safe and supportive environment for patient care by minimizing the risks associated with the use of medical equipment through inspection, preventive maintenance, and education of equipment users and maintainers. [Your facility's name] medical-equipment management program and management plan have been reviewed for content and scope. The medical-management plan was revised to reflect current (2004) standards and expectations.

Performance of program

The following chart shows the program objectives, the indicator(s) measured to achieve the stated objective(s), the effectiveness of the program, and future recommendations.

Indicators	Objectives	Performance (2001–2003)
Compliance rate of preventive maintenance (PM) activities for all items in medical-equipment program inventory	>/= 95% compliance rate 2001—93.8% compliance	(2001–2003) 2002—97.7% compliance 2003—98.4% compliance **Process stable; objective met**
Incident reporting: Equipment failures resulting in patient injury/negative outcome	No incidents of equipment failures resulting in injury/negative outcome	2001—0 incidents 2002—0 incidents 2003—0 incidents **Process stable; objective met**

Effectiveness of program/recommendations for improvement

The scope and performance of [your facility's name] medical-equipment program is determined to have been effective as called for in the 2003 management plan. This determination is based on a comprehensive evaluation of the medical-equipment management program and its objectives and monitoring of applicable performance indicators and the appropriate performance relative to objective goals, with improvement areas identified for ongoing monitoring. Additionally, no critical failure modes were identified as a function of the [your facility's name] incident-reporting system. The following improvement opportunities have been identified for 2004:

Improvement opportunity/objective	Indicator/measure
Compliance rate for PM activities—high-risk equipment	100% compliance rate (within 30 days of scheduled activity) for all high-risk medical equipment
Incidents resulting in patient injury/negative outcome	No incidents resulting in negative patient outcomes
Collaborate with education to improve equipment-management education efficiencies	Decrease in number of operator error findings (includes "could not duplicate" equipment-repair calls)

UTILITIES MANAGEMENT

Scope of program

[Your facility's name] utilities-management program provides a safe and supportive environment for patient care by minimizing the risks associated with using utility systems. The program does so by ensuring operational reliability, reducing the potential for healthcare–associated illnesses, mitigating the potential failure of utility systems, and educating utilities-systems end users and maintainers. [Your facility's name] utilities-management program and management plan have been reviewed for content and scope. The utilities-management plan was revised to reflect current (2004) standards and expectations.

Performance of program

The following chart shows the program objectives, the indicator(s) measured to achieve the stated objective(s), the effectiveness of the program, and future recommendations.

Indicators	Objectives	Performance (2001–2003)
Compliance rate of preventive-maintenance (PM) activities for all critical system components in the utilities-management program	>/= 95% compliance rate	2001—96% compliance rate 2002—97.5% compliance rate 2003—99.5% compliance rate **Process stable; objective met**
Incident reporting: Utility-system failures resulting in patient injury/negative outcome	No incidents of utility-system failures resulting in injury/negative outcome	2001—0 incidents 2002—0 incidents 2003—0 incidents **Process stable; objective met**

Effectiveness of program/recommendations for improvement

The scope and performance of [your facility's name] utility-systems program is determined to have been effective in the 2003 management plan. This determination is based on a comprehensive evaluation of the utility-systems management program and its objectives and monitoring of applicable performance indicators and performance relative to objective goals, with improvement areas identified for ongoing monitoring. Additionally, no critical failure modes were identified as a function of the [your facility's name] incident-reporting system. The following improvement opportunities have been identified for 2004:

Improvement opportunity/objective	Indicator/measure
Compliance rate for PM activities—high-risk equipment	100% compliance rate (within 30 days of scheduled activity) for all high-risk utility systems equipment
Incidents resulting in patient injury/negative outcome	No incidents resulting in negative patient outcomes
Collaborate with education to improve utility systems management education efficiencies	Decrease in number of operator error findings (includes "could not duplicate" utility-system trouble calls—19 reported in 2003)

APPENDIX:
FIVE FORMS FOR ONGOING EC EFFORTS

To further assist you in your efforts to produce an annual environment of care (EC) report to leaders, we've included five customizable tools in the appendix. They are

- a sample policy on new employee safety orientation. Use this policy to help guide your EC education efforts.

- a sample EC survey for employees. This survey should help you get a handle on employee knowledge and what areas may need further education.

- a sample workplace-violence checklist. From the Occupational Safety and Health Administration, this survey can help you identify potential workplace violence problems that you might want to address through EC performance-improvement projects.

- a sample checklist for clinical-alarm audibility. This checklist should help you comply with the Joint Commission on Accreditation of Healthcare Organizations' patient safety goal regarding clinical alarms.

- an emergency-management exercise evaluation form. Use this form to evaluate emergency-management drills and identify areas for improvement.

SAMPLE NEW EMPLOYEE SAFETY ORIENTATION

[Your facility's name] Medical Center

| SUBJECT: New employee safety orientation | MANUAL: Safety manual |
| | SECTION: |

I. Policy

All personnel who work at the hospital or at any hospital-sponsored, off-site clinics will receive a hospitalwide safety and environment of care orientation both to help them perform their job duties in accordance with the latest standards and to provide the highest level of service to patients.

II. Procedure

A. All new hospital employees will complete the safety/environment of care orientation on their first day of employment

B. Staff will receive an organizational and department-specific orientation that includes, as appropriate, information about
   1. general hospital safety
   2. electrical safety
   3. ergonomics
   4. security
   5. hazardous materials and waste management
   6. emergency management
   7. fire safety
   8. medical equipment
   9. utility management
   10. infection control
   11. quality-improvement activities
   12. organizational policies, procedures, and practices

C. Volunteers, contract personnel, physicians, and students will receive orientation as appropriate to their responsibilities

D. Training records will be maintained for four years after termination of employment

E. Annual refresher training will include both hospitalwide and department-specific topics

III. References

2004 JCAHO EC.1.10–9.10, HR.2.10–2.30

| ORIGINAL DATE: | SUPERSEDES: | PROC NO.: 3–3 |
| REVISION: DATE: | FILE NAME: | PAGE: 1 of 1 |

SAMPLE CHECKLIST FOR AUDIBILITY OF CLINICAL ALARMS

This checklist is one way to comply with the Joint Commission on Accreditation of Healthcare Organization's requirements for staff members to hear clinical alarms when they go off. This questionnaire is not all-inclusive, nor is it the only way to measure compliance for this National Patient Safety Goal. Your hospital will likely find other pertinent concerns to ask about as well.

* * *

Date: _____

Name: _____ Department: _____

Equipment/item tested (including model): _____

Manufacturer (if known): _____

Location of the equipment/item: _____

Day of the testing (e.g., Monday, Tuesday, etc.): _____

Time of the testing: _____

Was the alarm for the item on and working properly? Yes No

If no, please explain further: _____

Describe how far away you stepped from the equipment/item, and in each case, whether you could hear the alarm:

Distance: _____ Could you hear the alarm? _____

Distance: _____ Could you hear the alarm? _____

Distance: _____ Could you hear the alarm? _____

In cases where you couldn't hear the alarm, why was the alarm inaudible? _____
_____
_____
_____

Were there other noises competing with the clinical alarm (e.g., a paging system, nursing-station conversation, etc.)? _____
_____
_____

Is this equipment/item critical to patient care? Yes No

Do you have any suggestions for improvement? _____
_____
_____
_____

Source: The Joint Commission's Patient Safety Goals and the frequently asked questions section of its Web site (www.jcaho.org). John Rosing, FACHE, The Greeley Company, Marblehead, MA.

EMERGENCY-MANAGEMENT EXERCISE EVALUATION FORM

Date: _____   Exercise: _____

Unit/department being evaluated: _____

FACILITY

Place a check mark under the grade that best indicates your evaluation. (1 = lowest score; 5 = highest score)
(Your first test will establish a benchmark. Continuous improvement is the key.)

	1	2	3	4	5	N/A
Overhead announcement heard clearly?						
Fire doors operated properly?						
Fire pull-stations operable?						
Hallways cleared?						
Fire extinguishers located, charged, and dated properly?						

STAFF KNOWLEDGE

	1	2	3	4	5	N/A
Staff first-response actions?						
Staff knowledge of actions required?						
Supervisor advised and in charge?						
Patient-care actions exercised?						
Information reported from staff to supervisor?						
Staff knowledge of emergency-manual location?						
Staff use of emergency manual?						
Staff knowledge of evacuation or search process?						
Overall department/unit response?						

INCIDENT CONTROL

	1	2	3	4	5	N/A
Emergency operations center activated?						
Action log established?						
Labor pool established?						
Status information received, analyzed, and recorded?						
Exercise issues managed appropriately?						

Additional comments: _____

_____

_____

Overall exercise score for the department/unit evaluated: _____

When assigned to evaluate a hospital unit,

    1. question staff   2. observe actions   3. evaluate response

Evaluator: _____   Date completed: _____

WORKPLACE-VIOLENCE CHECKLIST

The checklist below offers an example of how hospitals might identify potential workplace violence problems. Designated, competent observers should make periodic inspections to evaluate workplace security hazards and threats of workplace violence. Schedule these inspections regularly, such as when new, previously unidentified security hazards are recognized; when occupational deaths, injuries, or threats of injury occur; and whenever workplace security conditions warrant an inspection.

Use the following checklist to identify and evaluate workplace security hazards. "True" answers indicate a potential risk for serious security hazards.

T ❑ F ❑ The hospital frequently confronts violent behavior and assaults on staff members.

T ❑ F ❑ Violence has occurred on the premises.

T ❑ F ❑ Patients, visitors, or coworkers assault, threaten, yell, push, or verbally abuse employees or use racist or sexist remarks.

T ❑ F ❑ Employees aren't required to report incidents or threats of violence, regardless of injury or severity, to their supervisors.

T ❑ F ❑ Employees haven't received training from the hospital to recognize and handle threatening, aggressive, or violent behavior.

T ❑ F ❑ Some managers, supervisors, or employees accept violence as part of the job.

T ❑ F ❑ The hospital doesn't restrict access and freedom of movement within the workplace to people who have legitimate reasons for being there.

T ❑ F ❑ The workplace security system is inadequate—for example, door locks malfunction, windows are not secure, and there are no physical barriers or containment systems.

T ❑ F ❑ Patients have assaulted, threatened, or verbally abused staff members.

T ❑ F ❑ The hospital hasn't offered medical and counseling services to employees who have been assaulted.

T ❑ F ❑ Alarm systems, such as panic alarm buttons, silent alarms, or personal electronic alarm systems, aren't used for prompt security assistance.

T ❑ F ❑ There is no regular training provided on the correct response to an alarm.

T ❑ F ❑ The hospital doesn't test security alarm systems on a monthly basis to ensure correct function.

T ❑ F ❑ The hospital doesn't employ security guards.

T ❑ F ❑ The hospital doesn't use closed-circuit cameras and mirrors to monitor dangerous areas.

T ❑ F ❑ Metal detectors aren't available or aren't used in the facility.

T ❑ F ❑ Employees haven't received training to recognize and control hostile and escalating behaviors, or to manage assaults.

T ❑ F ❑ Employees can't adjust work schedules to use the "buddy system" for visits to patients or visitors in areas where they feel threatened.

T ❑ F ❑ Communication services aren't available to staff members to enable them to request aid.

T ❑ F ❑ The hospital doesn't maintain its vehicles on a regular basis to ensure reliability and safety.

T ❑ F ❑ Employees work where assistance isn't readily available.

Source: The Occupational Safety and Health Administration's Hospital e-tool, available at www.osha.gov/SLTCetools/hospital/.

EMPLOYEE ENVIRONMENT OF CARE SURVEY

Please complete and return to the Safety Department.

Department: _____

1. **Can you describe the location of the fire exits nearest to your work area?**

   Yes   No   N/A

2. **Can you describe the nearest manual pull station to your work area?**

   Yes   No   N/A

3. **Can you describe the proper procedure for completing an incident report?**

   Yes   No   N/A

4. **If a visitor falls, is it appropriate to direct him or her to the Emergency Department for free treatment?**

   Yes   No   N/A

5. **Can you describe why red outlets are used?**

   Yes   No   N/A

6. **Are you familiar with the proper procedures for the reporting of defective nonmedical equipment?**

   Yes   No   N/A

7. **Can you describe the purpose of Material Safety Data Sheets (MSDS)?**

   Yes   No   N/A

8. **Can you describe how to obtain a chemical's MSDS?**

   Yes   No   N/A

9. **Can you describe how you know when a piece of medical equipment was last inspected?**

   Yes   No   N/A

10. **Can you describe the process for reporting defective medical equipment?**

    Yes   No   N/A

11. **Can you describe how to access the Disaster Plans?**

    Yes   No   N/A

12. **Do you know how to report an incident of workplace violence?**

    Yes   No   N/A

13. **Do you know how to access information and resources if you experience workplace violence?**

    Yes   No   N/A